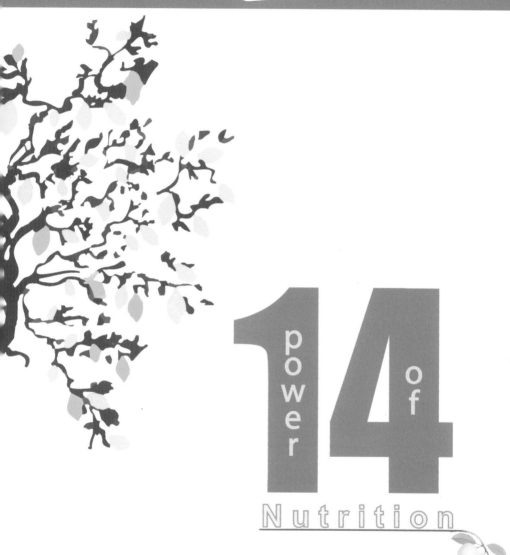

# power 14 of

## Nutrition

# By Anthony McClanahan

The supplements, vitamins, and food information contained in this book are based on Anthony McClanahan's experiences, research, personal and professional experiences. They are in no way a substitute for consulting with your physician or health-care providers. The author does not advocate the use of any particular health-care protocol, but believes the information in this book can help the general public become healthier. If the reader has any question regarding health concerns, the author strongly suggests consulting a professional health-care advisor.

The opinions expressed in this manuscript are solely the opinions of the author and do not represent the opinions or thoughts of the publisher. The author has represented and warranted full ownership and/or legal right to publish all the materials in this book.

"Where you start is not nearly as important as where you finish." – Zig Ziglar

This book is dedicated to my Grandma and Grandpa Marion for sharing the fruits of their beautiful garden with the entire community. Sharing is caring. *The Power of 14* is dedicated to you.

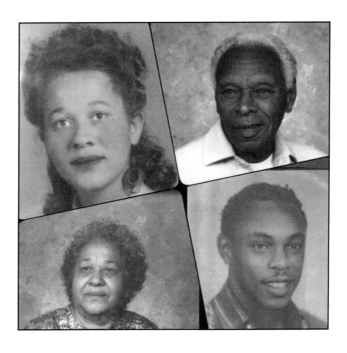

# Table of Contents

Why It All Started ........................................................ i

Testimonial from Lori..................................................... v

Preface .................................................................... vii

Testimonial from Tim and Mandi ...................................... xii

Introduction: Here's How It Works! ................................... 1

Success of a Four-Quarter Athlete .................................... 5

Testimonial from Trina .................................................. 8

Bubble.................................................................... 10

Blue 41. Set Go!........................................................ 13

Testimonial from Ty ..................................................... 15

Understanding Protein.................................................. 18

Testimonial from Maureen.............................................. 27

14 Supplements (vitamins and minerals that will
      fire up your fat-burning program)................................ 29

14 "Energy" Foods That Will Supercharge Your Body! .............. 32

14 Creative Ways to Simplify Your Plan.............................. 34

Blue Print to Excellence: 14 Weight Loss Metabolism
      Boosting Dishes................................................... 38

Testimonial from Sandy ............................................... 44

Power of 14 Journal.................................................... 47

The Power of 14 Shopping List........................................ 48

Shopping List – Week 1 ............................................... 49

14 Days to Success – Week 1 ......................................... 50

Shopping List – Week 2 ............................................... 67

14 Days to Success – Week 2 ......................................... 68

Acknowledgements .................................................... 85

Sources.................................................................. 86

Together we will take a journey that will
transform every aspect of your life.
To the top we go. Drive hard, my friends.
~ Anthony McClanahan, #41

Enjoy the Power of 14!

# Why It All Started

In life, something very traumatic has to happen in order for change to take place. This happened to me in 1998 when I suffered a blow to my neck during a game while playing football for the Calgary Stampeders. It was November 14, we were playing Saskatchewan Roughriders, another team in the Canadian Football League. During the play I received an injury to my neck. The injury I sustained from this tackle caused my C4 - C6 to tear from an impact of what felt like a thousand pounds of elephant strength placing pressure to my head which caused me to blackout. As I lay on the football field in front of 45,000 people in Calgary, Alberta, I lost complete movement of my left side for about five minutes. When I finally realized I wasn't completely paralyzed, I stood up with the help of my teammates. On the sidelines, my coaches asked me if I was okay. Knowing the expectations of a football player I was determined to regain my composure, cowboy up, and get back in the game. At the time I did not realize that it would be the biggest life-changing mistake I would ever make. I continued to play injured for seven more weeks, all the while hiding my pain. I overcompensated for my left side by hitting with my right shoulder until I suddenly began to show signs of weakness. At that point, I decided to tell someone I was seriously injured and needed help. Soon enough I was having surgery.

The doctors filmed my surgery experience for a medical documentary. The entire surgery from the time I was given the anesthesia to completion was sixteen hours. In order to complete the operation on my neck, doctors used a cadaver bone and placed a titanium plate over the C4-C5 disc to fuse them together, a procedure that was very painful. My road to recovery was long and hard. I spent the rest of the season on the sideline, thankful we still ended up winning the 1998 Grey Cup. The following season I signed with the Saskatchewan Roughriders. With my neck still so unstable, I decided to end my football career. If it wasn't for my aggressive consumption of protein in my diet, I may not be where my physical health is today. I have always included three to four shakes per day and taken high doses of vitamin C, magnesium, zinc, selenium, chromium, and amino acids in addition to my meal-planning routine. My diet would consist of raw vegetables, chicken, turkey, fish, nuts, and fruits that were green. I remember my grandmother telling me that eating green and lean was the way to rid the toxins from your body. She also suggested that whey protein was a natural pain remedy. That was some thirty-five years ago, and now similar information is found all over the Internet. How did she know that? The Power of 14 started with my grandmother, Clara Marion. I knew that in order to overcome my pain and become strong again I had to heal myself, especially because I have never been big on taking any sort of medication. After several months of self-healing and strengthening my body again, I decided to venture into the world of sports entertainment.

I traveled to LA and was able to land a gig with the hit television show *Battledome*, produced by Sony Pictures. During the filming of one of the shows, I took a fall that re-injured my neck for the second time and caused me to regress in my healing. Again, I refused therapy and continued a regimen of detoxing, cleansing, and using several nutritional supplements. I stayed completely true to my lifestyle of eating clean and green. Even though my neck could not withstand impact sports any longer, I still had my health and a hard body with a super-high endurance level. My grandmother always said, "Nutrition was the answer, not the pain meds." She would feed me and the entire local community from her garden. There she grew a variety of 14 fruits and vegetables.

She called it her "Garden of Eden." I promised her that I would one day feed people just as she did. I would take the number 14 and make it a health and fitness brand and share it with the entire world. Once again I took her advice. This helped me heal faster and I came back stronger!

The Power of 14 was designed to help speed up the conventional medical treatments and safely but greatly improve their effectiveness. I knew that the pills prescribed could cause harm to my body, but using the right nutritional supplements, eating green, and keeping other foods low in fat would help me get moving again. Many people have conquered such things as cancer, pain, and injuries by following this example. I knew that by educating people with the proper nutrition needed daily, I could also help change their physique. As a trainer I began to test this philosophy on my clients. Within a couple of days all my clients and I noticed significant weight loss for those following the plan. Knowing this combined with having pain all my athletic life and choosing to be on a strict eating plan influenced me to write this book. Since I was a linebacker and traditionally they wear higher numbers, I was not able to wear number 14 on my jersey. By flipping the number to 41, I still felt like I was honoring my grandma and it became my superhero safety mechanism! As long as I have #41 she is close to me.

From my grandma's garden I came up with the slogan "Power of 14," which in turn helped me to create my company name, 41 Sports. My grandma helped nourish a lot of people over many years, and now it is my turn to carry forth her traditions and help some really important people like you! She did!

"To listen to your mind is
success waiting to happen."
The Power of 14 is a way of life! Own it.
Anthony McClanahan, #41

# Testimonial from Lori

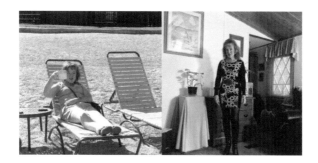

41, you are amazing and I cannot thank you enough! My weight has yo-yoed all my life and I have been on every diet and exercise plan out there, I was almost 300 lbs at my heaviest. August 10, 2010 I was involved in a head-on 80 mph impact collision that crushed my feet. The doctors at that time did not know if I was going to ever walk again, but I did. I started my new journey in a wheelchair at 5'4", 154 lbs, then after I got rid of the walking boots and the cane I was peer-pressured into joining 41 Sports Boot Camp in late 2011. My mobility was still not very good and I did not believe I could do it, let alone keep up. I had no confidence and doubted it would do any good as the doctors told me I would never be able to run. I just wanted to firm/tone up (did not think it was possible) and lose a little weight. WOW! I did not expect to ever be where I am today and never ever thought I would continue! *Not long after joining 41 Sports and following the food plan, I was 143 lbs. My dream/fantasy weight was 135 lbs but 41 said 130 lbs – I laughed! I could not believe I went from size 9/10 to a size 4 regular. This blew my mind and I started to wholeheartedly believe in 41 and his program. I am a huge skeptic, but I continued and started his Pro Grade products and*

*did 41's eating plan. I trained with 41 Sports as well. It was then that I started seeing real results, and one night I went shopping since I needed new clothes and I would be shopping for a size 2! I cried.... size 2!!!! A very fit not sick 2! I am almost 52 years old and have never felt this good!* I can now keep up with my 3 grandkids; I sleep better and have way more energy. In 3/2013, I did my first 5k in 31 minutes, and on 4/20/13 I ran a 5k in 29 minutes. My next goal is a 10k so watch out, here I come! I have also not had a cold or flu in 2 years, maybe a little under-the-weather day, but that is it! I also love the Krill Oil & the Fusion drink. Love you & Thank you, 41!!! My 28-year-old Baby Belly is gone and I am now 128 lbs. 41 Sports has changed my life! I am very proud to say I am **41 Strong** today and plan to keep it that way!!!

# Preface

As the days, weeks, then years go by, I often wonder what changes may lie ahead that will affect my life as I know it. As people in a fast-paced society, we take advantage of life until an unexpected event makes us evaluate life as we know it. These events can range from losing a loved one to our own health issues. Either way, in order to continue we must take a look at our own life and make major changes to our lifestyles. There is no way to tell if and when a day like this will come, so why not just enjoy every day as if it was your last. The best way to do this is to train, eat healthy, and enjoy life. Drive hard to the top! Never look back. Set Go!

First, I want to say thank you for believing in me and my expertise. My motivation for writing this book is to help people like you change their lives for the better by eating healthier and training daily. You will become stronger than you ever imagined. I am so excited you have decided to take this journey with me. I have to ask, because I say this over and over, if you have no beginning or significant reason to take care of your mind, body, and soul, then you will not have the intrinsic desire to stick with and change your ways. Let's begin by asking yourself: Do I really need to get off that couch and workout? Is it possible that my neighbor truly has a magic pill and it will help me to shed twenty pounds before that next vacation? What if they did and you lost that weight? Would you be any healthier and stronger than before the pill? The answer is simple. NO! Who are you kidding? It is more important to eat healthy and train hard just like your kids or grandkids who run faster and have more energy than you do. Maybe your doctor has said every year to shed some weight but you keep gaining and now your heart is on its last beat or you are pre-diabetic.

Ask yourself, what is the use of training hard daily and eating healthy? As a trainer, I have heard every excuse known to man on why most people (like one-third of the world) never take time to work on themselves, and the ones that do only go for a short period of time and quit. One of the worst times is at New Year's with all the weight loss resolutions that begin and fail on this day. The first of the year is not a time to even mention weight loss. Why sabotage yourself? How about we modify our days and take each one of them slowly? How about we design a workout system you can do on a busy schedule? How about we prepare our foods on Sunday and pack them to last for a few days? Why not sweat and have a bit of pain? How about you stop making excuses and start asking questions on how to have better health? See, it's okay to hurt. It's okay to have a little pain. It's okay to eat foods that are not the best choice for you in moderation. The goal is to get on a plan and stick with it. There is no such thing as a cheat day; people fall off the plan and don't get back on track. There will always be an "event." I will teach you to prepare ahead of time and plan for what you can enjoy at these "events." Do not let them turn your hard work into excuses and poor choices. Plan your day. Morning workouts are the best, leaving no time for an excuse! Make it a habit of getting up at 5:30 am and busting your butt to make an impact on your health and fitness. The **Power of 14** is for everyone. If you want to become confident and take back that sexy attitude and body to boogie in, then bring it daily. Oh, and if that word "old" comes out of your mouth, find a new one to say. OLD is the new young. Even if you can't run you can have the "**Power of 14**." As long as you have a heart, you can train! Ready? Set Go! Drive hard to the top! Never look back. Get out that pen and get ready to take some notes. I mean workout daily and plan your meals like it's never been done. You have nothing holding you back. Bring it!

> Former Washington State Head Coach Mike Price once said, "McClanahan, you play the game of football like a relentless beast." Now, I train like one. Set Go! – #41

Working out has always been a part of my life. In fact, I cannot remember a time that I did not train. I can remember training as far back as age three, and that has set the stage for my career as professional athlete and now fitness professional. It started by being pulled in a wagon by my dad, Brent McClanahan, and running side by side with him as much as possible at a very young age. Dad, at the time, played football for the Minnesota Vikings. I remember his philosophy was to be fit in the off-season so when it was time for preseason camp he would be physically ready to go, and then at the start of the season, he would not hurt so badly. Sure enough, what he said was true and I found out soon enough with a lifetime of playing football. I dedicated myself to training in the early mornings. I would get up and get my day started before going to school and run for miles both during the season and off-season. While running on the streets of Bakersfield, California, I would also stop and perform 500 sit-ups, 300 pushups, and 200 jumping jacks. These drills were also performed by the late Walter Payton, and players like Herschel Walker and Ronnie Lott while playing professional football. It seemed like the players from the 1970s and early 1980s were driven to be champions and they knew exactly what to do in order to be the best. Since I wanted to also perform at the elite level and this training helped them to be the best, I figured it would certainly help me to take my athleticism to the top level also. See, it takes a person with a strong heart and desire to excel to be able to wake up each morning, get out of bed, and go train in 20-degree weather and workout outside. Someone has to have a huge understanding of their inner self and their limitless ability to achieve their dreams one day at a time. *It takes Heart. It takes Dedication. It takes believing in yourself when no one else does.* You have to want to achieve greatness in your fitness and health. It has to be done for you and you alone.

As much as I would like to tell you about my fitness routine and all the boot camps and private training 41 has done over the years, I can honestly say it's not important at this time, but it is important. What is important right now is that you pick up a glass of water and a pen and begin to read and make notes inside your **Power of 14 Program Guide**. The **Power of 14** is all you will ever need in your life. It doesn't matter if you are a professional bodybuilder, retired pro athlete or a stay-at-home mom; over time we all need a coach or someone to hold you accountable. They say you can't teach an old dog new tricks; when you give up on the old dog, he simply quits. The **Power of 14** is easy to follow and understand. It will allow you to take baby steps along your journey. I will be available to you for support because there is no quitting allowed. See, maintaining my health and fitness has been lifelong and my family and friends know this. The more successful my clients are, the more my longtime friends are turning to me for help. They too are succeeding with the **Power of 14**. This is my dream, to be able to teach those I care about how to live a healthy lifestyle in order to fully be able to enjoy their life. They usually want to know how to get in shape. Shocked of course, I can never imagine getting out of shape and not eating healthy every day to stay in the best shape of my life. I can remember being in the locker room of the Calgary Stampeders, I would keep inside my locker the daily outfit: helmet, shoulder pads, mouthpiece, "football stuff," and a blender to make shakes. Yes, a blender and tons of supplements. Every day before practice and film, I would make a shake. As a matter of fact, after practice and an ice bath, I would blend a second shake. Funny thing is all the guys would say, "41, you are nuts." Now the same guys are calling asking me for help. The **Power of 14** is a lifestyle, not a diet. Over time as you see your body change and energy level increase with this program, you will experience a winning attitude. You will have more drive and stamina to live your life. See, the top is beautiful and with the proper coaching, technique, and a plan, anyone can be a success story.

Drive Hard to The Top!
Anthony McClanahan, #41

# Testimonial from Tim and Mandi

## Tim Atkins, 31

I've been a police officer for 7 years in Washington State, and upon opening up my own insurance agency, I had to move to a reserve position in my department. I worked at a desk day in and day out, and over the course of 2 years I gained over 70 pounds without even realizing it. I was tired all of the time, and always felt sick. I had a background of bodybuilding when I was in my early 20's; I never thought I'd gain weight like that. One night while on patrol, I noticed my heart was beating rapidly, and I was involved in a foot pursuit shortly thereafter. I could hardly keep up running to chase after the suspect. Needless to say, my heart issues and health issues scared me and I knew it was time to make the change. I started

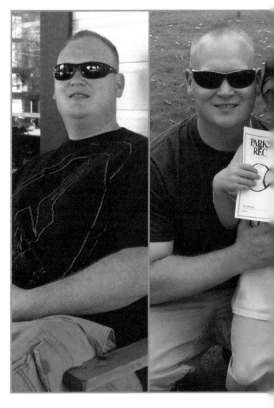

working with Anthony in April of 2013, and immediately started seeing results by using his nutrition plan and workouts. I entered his program weighing in at 288 pounds, at 6'1", and within 8 months I was down to 225 pounds. I met the goals we set at the beginning, and now I am currently working towards new ones.

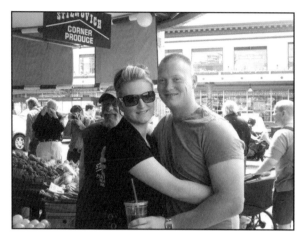

*Tim and Mandi Atkins*

## Mandi Atkins, 29

I have never had a "weight problem" in my entire life, up until I had my 3rd baby. In January 2010, after having my daughter, I weighed in at 196 pounds. By March, after doing everything I knew to do, I still weighed 180 pounds. I am 5'7", with a normally smaller frame that holds weight evenly. I was very frustrated. I battled on through the summer and only managed to lose about 10 more pounds, despite my

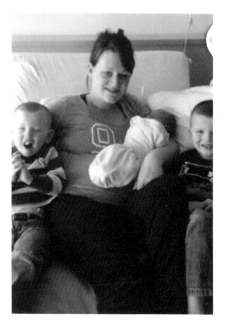

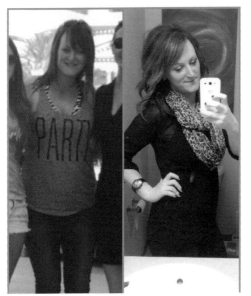

strongest efforts to lose more. My husband had lost a ton of weight following Anthony's program, so I decided it was time for me to do the same. I entered Anthony's program September of 2013 at 169 pounds, shoving myself into a size 10. Today, February of 2014, I am at 137 pounds, and easily fitting into a size 6. I have lost the weight I wanted; now my focus is on building muscle and endurance. I am in better shape than I was the day I got married, even after 3 babies in a short 5-year span. I continue to follow the lifestyle eating plan that I started last year with Anthony; it is really just my new way of living!

# Introduction: Here's How It Works!

*The Power of 14* is a self-help workbook journal that will challenge you to be the best you can be. This book will encourage you when you need it the most. It will keep you honest on those challenging days when you just don't have time to eat or work towards your goals. The Power of 14 is a program that will not allow you to cheat on your meals or workouts.

As in any successful program, there has to be a regimen to follow. Without a regimen we are aimlessly trying to achieve results without the necessary information. How do you get where you want to go without a plan to get there? As a professional athlete, without a regimen during the season, football players are useless. So, on the first day of training camp, we are given a schedule to follow that takes us to the end of the year. In this schedule it outlines film study, treatment times, media, training table, workout, etc. Once this schedule is in our hands, it gives the players opportunity to balance home life with the training schedule of a professional athlete. The time required by the NFL/CFL typically consumes an average of well over eight hours a day of commitment to the team and training. This leaves very little time to prepare meals on the job. Food consumption many times must occur in the locker room. In order to maintain optimal health to play at the professional level, the guys had to care about their health and had to consume only foods high in nutrients to gain the most energy and stamina in a day. In order to do this they would consume shakes and eat prepared healthy meals about every two to three hours. The Power of 14 will show you how to eat and shed weight while doing it. As professional athletes, we would have to eat or drink a protein shake just to keep up the calories for weight maintenance, and more so for any weight gain to occur. The Power of 14 will help you to stay dedicated to transforming your body and mind while consuming foods and drinking fluids every two to three hours a day like athletes. Of course this journey is not a weight-gain journey; the Power of 14 will teach you how to shed the unwanted fat and in time help you achieve the goals you want to achieve. This program will teach you to eat to live and not starve yourself, all the while detoxifying your body and giving it proper nutrition to form the foundation needed to build a stronger body. Point being is the Power of 14 will help you organize your daily schedule.

This program is not just about buying a book and going at it alone. This program will walk you through the first two weeks to assure maximum results. The Power of 14 and I, 41, will coach you every step of the way. The first program is 14 days. Most programs target 90 days to success, and during this time most people lose interest. With the Power of 14, you will see results in the first week, which will keep you motivated. For a fun motivator, have someone take some "before" pictures of you. Then along the way and definitely when you reach your goal, take more photos! On the Power of 14 an average person loses 2-6 lbs per week. The only thing I need from you is to weigh at the beginning, middle, and end of the 14 days in order to track your weight loss – no more, no less. Please do not get on the scale daily. Follow the plan exactly because the Power of 14 will help you take the steps you need to succeed.

When the game is on the line in football, if you don't execute a prepared play, you jeopardize your chance of success. The same needs to happen in order to have a greater chance of success at your new way of eating. You have to be prepared and follow the plan. On the Power of 14, you will have to eat and drink something with nutritional value every 2.5 hours. The Power of 14 will be all about the choices you make every day, at every meal, in order to make the change. It's time for a transformation to occur. The Power of 14 is a complete lifestyle change. I want you to begin to eat normal and healthy to reach your goals of having a lean look. You will find you are a much happier person with the right amount of food and nutrition. If you are ever having a hard time following the plan and need any type of coaching support, contact 41. On this long journey you will have access to 41's e-mail address and the private Facebook group page. On this page you will be able to share your success stories and seek extra food coaching and/or program support. The Power of 14 will show you how to win. 41 will help you stay driven and hold you accountable. Let's win with the Power of 14.

As a champion linebacker, I can honestly say it took help from my team and everyone that played a vital part in my life to win a championship. This program is also all about team, and over the course of this journey you will hear lots of terms, many football references, to help you achieve your goals using what I like to call "The Bubble." The Bubble is the place you will go to find answers and peace all in one place. The Bubble will be your team in the locker room. We will discuss more of The Bubble later.

Get ready to have success with the Power of 14. As we work on this journey together, simply know all you need is a plan of attack. The Power of 14 is the tool needed to make your lifestyle change, and it works alongside your day-to-day schedule. The Power of 14 will help you shed the weight you are looking to drop each and every week. No counting of calories, no phony promises. This is a good old-fashioned way of doing hard work. Like my Grandmother Marion always said on Sunday to prepare me for the week, "If you win daily in the kitchen, it will help you to win on the field." Grandmother Marion knew that nutrition was an important part of sports performance and our overall health. So as long as you make a plan with 41 using the POWER OF 14, be prepared to win!

The Power of 14 is truly the only
way to accomplish superior goals.
You must follow your heart to reach the top!
Set Go! Drive hard to the top
and never look back!
Anthony McClanahan, #41

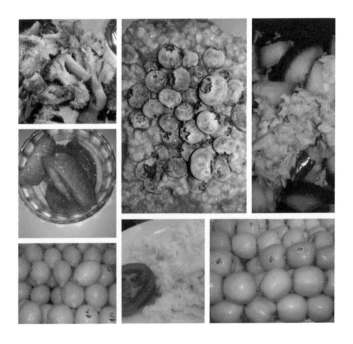

# Success of a
# Four-Quarter Athlete

The last thing one would probably expect was to be sitting here reading a program designed by a football player turned fitness guru. Who would have thought such a thing? Especially when most athletes that retire from professional sports eat whatever they want and they usually leave the training for the younger generation. There are many reasons why, but know that I watched my grandparents exhibit such a passion towards maintaining their own health in order to support the family and community in sports that it lit a flame in me that burns bright enough for everyone. This flame instilled in me explains the Power of 14 and why so many of my clients have made health and fitness a vital part of their lives. They dedicate themselves to training and eating off the Power of 14 food list. The Power of 14 is a four-quarter program that has to be followed 100% to have the ultimate weight-loss success. Meaning when it says green apples, red is not okay. Just like playing in a game of football, it takes success in all four quarters to win the game. So in each quarter you have to give 100% in order to have complete weight-loss success. You have to keep the flame alive.

I am laughing out loud now from being the linebacker I used to be. The one who played relentless and at any cost, the one who would take down an offensive lineman to help the rest of the defense tackle an opponent, the linebacker now turned fitness guru! Yes, I do expect you to read the entire program and journal your hearts out and win. See it's all about being visual, being direct, having passion, and the only way you stay motivated is to **Taste It, Breathe It, Smell It,** and **Live It**. Our internal fire, that flame flickering, is only turned up when something makes us excited. Each week you are to weigh in and share with a family member or someone you have placed on your team to win. This process will help take you to the top!

So what do I mean when I say **Taste It, Breathe It, Smell It, and Live It**?

**Taste It:** With the right amount of commitment you will "taste" what it is like to feel better and look better. After the "taste," will you have what it takes to stick to it and reach your goal and then begin another?

**Breathe It:** Can you block out all of your current issues and check the many excuses you make daily in your life into the locker room? Use your internal drive to get the same mindset of an athlete who is set out to win by creating positive habits before a game. They may say out loud to themselves, inside the locker room, "Self, today nothing bothers me, today is my day!" Once you conquer your emotions, YOU WIN!

**Smell It:** I can remember walking into the locker room for practice and the smell giving me confidence that I could do anything and would run out onto the field daily with my head held high. You too need to smell your success. How can one win if you have no power? 41 wants you to smell power, success, and life. The four team rules to success will help while you are in a group of people for dinner and they are all picking on you because you are choosing not to eat fatty foods. Simply remember to smell your success, keep your fire burning. You're on the Power of 14 and it speaks for itself. Show those around you that you have an ambition to win.

**Live It:** For all the things you dream to happen, you must live by higher standards. If we are to win, we must plan and continue to seek positive and creative things. This also means we must place ourselves around positive and supportive people. If you want to have success with the Power of 14, you must live by it and for it. Can you smell victory? Live for you and never let anyone tell you it's a waste of time. Over the years, I have heard every excuse possible on why someone wanted to stop shedding weight after losing 40 lbs, knowing they had 60 lbs to go. One excuse that comes to mind is, "My husband/wife likes me at this weight just fine." Stop! This is about you and your health. Without a plan, a year from now you will find you have gained more weight and now have even more to lose. I want to help you break the cycle. Once you start a program, take it to the end and continue to stay on a lifestyle plan that fits you, not someone else. Team rules are important. **LET'S WIN!**

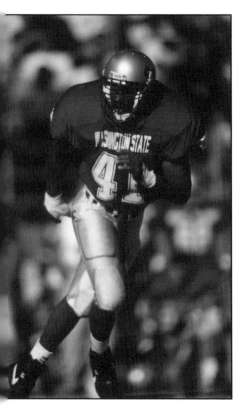

Never give up! No matter what you do in life, someone is always watching. So, always give 100% effort at everything you do. – #41

# Testimonial from Trina

Anthony McClanahan of 41 Sports Fitness Boot Camps changed my life. It was 5 1/2 years ago that a friend of mine told me about one of the defensive coaches of our son's high school football team. He was starting a 5:30 am boot camp. I was so excited! When I was in high school I tried out for the basketball team, and was cut! Over the last 30 years I have had so many gym memberships that were a total waste of money! So, I was very excited about this boot camp! I was not impressed with the time of 5:30 in the morning but after the first 3 weeks of boot camp,

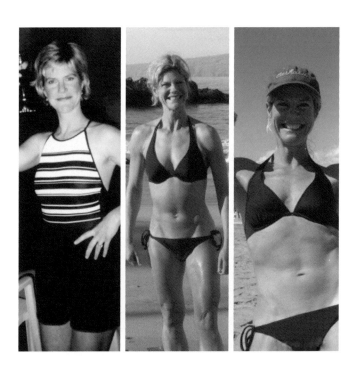

I lost weight, inches, gained energy, strength, endurance, mental health, and wonderful friends! Anthony called me personally and told me how much weight and inches I lost and then told me I was a natural athlete! I broke into tears! I'm an ATHLETE!!!! For the first time in my life, I felt like I was a part of a team! Anthony McClanahan takes us on amazing adventures every day! 41 Adventures Boot Camp is an outdoor boot camp that meets all over Whatcom County.

The food and fitness program has changed my life forever! He has taken us on mud runs, running mountains and marathons, swimming in the bay, working out in lakes, hiking in the woods, climbing ropes, running with planks, running hills with rocks, 1,000 abs in 17 minutes, and the best Booty Jam ever!! Anthony is the greatest trainer, motivator, and has become a great friend to me and my family. I'm a morning person now. I love to wake up at 5:30 am and start my day with 41 Sports!!!

# Bubble

It is no secret that the reason we need a bubble is because we are all on an emotional roller-coaster ride trying to strive to be the best we can be. Any time we attempt a new program to lose weight, we start off with the best of intentions, but because we have not found our inner bubble, external influences challenge us beyond our inner strength.

The Power of 14 will help you with your roller coaster. The bubble is the place I want you to go when you need to relax, seek guidance, strength, or just peace of mind. This is the little place you can go to and hide to refocus your mind and spirit; the bubble. You need to create a space in your mind where you can focus on your goal and how good it will feel to be on top, to conquer your desire to be healthier, leaner, and sexier. This is your bubble and no one is allowed into your bubble. This is the place you shut everyone out and you focus only on you. Your bubble holds both the good and the ugly. One of the major subject areas in your bubble will be your emotions. This journey will be an emotional one with all the major success you will have

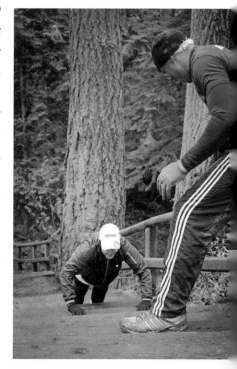

in your weight loss. Your emotions will run high and low and you need your bubble to cope with both. Use your bubble daily. Many major-league pitchers have gone to the bubble to block out the fan-base noise in the stadium when the game was on the line, helping them to throw that perfect pitch. The bubble is your golden egg machine. Place your goal inside your bubble, such as wanting to fit into a sexy dress for a special occasion. Then think, what do I need to do to reach this goal using the Power of 14? Is there an area on my body I need to focus on that is associated with this reward? Maybe you would say back and arms. Place it in the bubble and do whatever it takes to win. You are now well within your bubble and it's time to explore a new you. One thing 41 enjoys is bringing a reward to the bubble. Reward yourself each week you successfully use your bubble. Once you get that sexy back you can take self-esteem to the top!

"Did you know that if you fail at one thing, you have a chance to pick up and do it even better the next time it comes around. Failure is a good thing because it challenges you and makes us stronger. So the next time you run out of steam training hardcore or are stuck on a project, challenge yourself and bring it! Remember you're only letting down yourself if you give up. Sometimes we fail, sometimes we win! But if you never give up, you will succeed!"
Drive hard to the top! ~ #41

# Blue 41. Set Go!

As you begin your journey with the Power of 14, give it your all. Get into your bubble and put forth 100% effort at everything you do. Blue 41. Set Go! Continue to have a mindset to hold nothing back so you gain the most with the effort you put forth. When you train, push yourself to failure, and when you prepare your meals for the week, make sure you follow through with the plan after the prep. So what are you waiting for? Get out your pen and let's begin your journey to the top! Before we begin, I just want to remind you to have fun. This program by no means should make you stressed out. **The things that happen to you daily in your life should not reflect the foods you do or do not choose to eat. The Power of 14 is about your lifestyle change. At the end of the day you still have to live, and the only way is to get the proper nutrition.** For an example, a lady was on her way to drop her daughter off at the airport, and along the way she got a phone call that her other daughter was in the emergency room. Twelve hours later she still hadn't eaten or drank anything. I understand there are life-changing experiences and emergencies that can cause one not to worry about oneself and cause the plan to be completely nonexistent. However, an emergency or a situation should not cause a person to stop taking care of themselves. At the end of the day the person she was trying to take care of was fine, but she was not. Twelve hours into her day she was admitted to the hospital due to dehydration, lack of food, and stress. Remember to stay the course and continue on the journey. The Power of 14 will teach you to keep foods on you at all times.

We are only as strong as our weakest link. Drive hard to the top!

So here we are at the bottom of the hill trying to decide if we sprint to the top or slowly jog. The Power of 14 has a plan for you. It is time to determine if you have a strong work ethic and are dedicated and willing to have fun. My belief is when you are enjoying what you do and believe in yourself, the fun just comes naturally. So now you have the opportunity to start the Power of 14! What measures will you take to better yourself? Can you go that extra mile to complete your task? Can you set a few goals and accomplish them? I think you can. Get up and tell yourself I will strive to be better than yesterday. The Power of 14 will completely change you. It will give you confidence to achieve and believe in yourself like never before. Over the next 14 days we are going to have the most amazing journey together. After 14 days the journey will continue for those with the heart and passion to succeed. Let's have some fun out there, people. Please enjoy the adventure.

# Ty

Why am I breathing hard after I tie my shoes? Oh that's right, I'm fat and I'm squishing myself when bending over. Okay, time to do something about it because I'm not going to be the dad at the pool 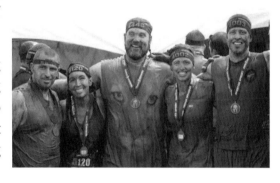 wearing a t-shirt in the water. Granted I'm not looking for a 6 pack…well I am but a 6 pack of Busch Light, but I want to get myself right. About a year and a half ago my dad went to the doctor and they told him that if he walked back out the door he came in, diabetes was waiting at the truck. My dad made a decision to get some help and he lost 90 lbs in approx. 8 months. Of course he hired a nutritionist, a therapist, a psychologist, and a trainer. He was spending approx. $2K/mo. for help. I didn't want this same discussion with my doctor so I reached out to my good friend and fellow Coug Anthony. I met him years ago through a mutual friend and he always had a ton of energy and is seriously the most cut-up 40-year-old dude I've ever seen. I knew he ran boot camps, but had no idea about his online training. I reached out via Facebook just to see if he could write a plan for me and he let me know all about his online training regimen…exactly what I was looking for!

Anthony and I went over goals and some realistic expectations.

One goal I had was that I just signed up for the Spartan Race that was in approx. 8 months. Anthony wrote me a day-by-day food plan and gave me a handful of workouts that I could do at home in only about 30 minutes. Most of them were 5–8 minute videos on YouTube that I would go 4 quarters of this workout. It was awesome because I could set up my iPad in the garage and go!

My biggest issue was the accountability. Anthony did an awesome job of texting me 2–3 times a day about my eating and what workout I completed. I never wanted to disappoint him (or myself) and I knew those texts were coming. I was an athlete through high school and part of college, so the workouts weren't the toughest part. It was the eating. I had gotten into such a habit of fast food because I'm always on the go and it was slowly killing me. Anthony did a great job of educating me on food, portion control, and planning! He made it specific to me, so it was helping with the workouts. Trust me, there were more days than not, I wanted to throw my phone when his text came through or when I KNEW I had to get my workout in because when I weighed myself at the end of the week there's no way I could gain. He got me in a rhythm to where even when I had some trips planned (Vegas and California), I PLANNED! I knew what I was going to do and I knew I wanted to have a steak and my favorite place and have a drink…or 10. But I let Anthony know and we planned around that. I did my workouts in the hotel gym, we planned major walks every day, and I knew what drinks I could and couldn't have. This planning had me either continuing to lose or maintain…there was no gain through my vacations. That made the day to day at home that much easier. It wasn't anything outrageous. My workouts moved to approx. 45 minutes, maybe an hour because I was running more, but nothing that I couldn't get done after the kids went to bed or before they got up in the AM. My meals changed too. Right as my body would be used to something and plateau, he mixed it up.

Anthony was right there with me the whole time. Jump to 7 months of this and I went from 6'4", 311 lbs to 6'4", 244 lbs... yup, 67 lbs and I completed that Spartan.

41 Sports and Anthony are the real deal. He changed my life and put some years back on. Thank you, 41 Sports, and GO COUGS!

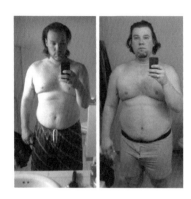

*Ty*

# Understanding Protein

When you think of protein intake with the Power of 14, realize it works to help decrease appetite and control the amount of calories you are taking in. While you are on the Power of 14, never count your caloric intake because we eat to burn. That means when you're hungry, you eat from the plan. Research has proven that eating the right foods when hungry will actually help reduce your body fat. The Power of 14 believes in taking in daily amounts of protein to support your body's needs to maintain lean muscle mass, help with training recovery, support cell development and tissue growth. While on the Power of 14, your "diet" will help control blood fats and create lean muscle. I say this lightly because this is a new way of eating, not a diet.

While I was playing football I often got hungry, and if I consumed a bit of protein before practice or a game the hungry feeling went away. I called it my fuel supply since protein and "diet" has been very tricky to research. We do know that in order to keep our brain functioning properly, we need to have fewer insulin spikes and keep our blood sugar levels balanced. We need to consume more protein in our daily diet to win.

## How to Calculate Your Protein Needs:

1. Weight in pounds divided by 2.2 = weight in kg
2. Weight in kg x 0.8 - 1.8 gm/kg = protein gm

Use a lower number if you are in good health and are sedentary (i.e., 0.8). Use a higher number (between 1 and 1.8) if you are under stress, pregnant, recovering from an illness, or if you are involved in consistent and intense weight or endurance training.

Example:   154 lb male who is a regular exerciser and lifts weights

154 lbs / 2.2 = 70 kg
70 kg x 1.5 = 105 gm protein/day

## Calculating Protein as a Percentage of Total Calories:

Another way to calculate how much protein you need is by using daily calorie intake and the percentage of calories that will come from protein. To do this, you'll need to know how many calories your body needs each day.

"Protein is essential to the development of muscle growth and even more so while losing weight. Take control of your destiny. Drive hard to the Top!"

During my football days, the following list of foods made up my daily diet. They helped me to stay strong when playing football, and when I was injured these are the foods that helped me to recover quickly. These foods are filled with proteins and amino acids that will jumpstart your healthy transformation. They always say eating healthy costs more; not true, when you have a plan it actually will save you money in the long run. The Power of 14 will take you back to your optimum health.

"Did you know that plant foods contain the same eight amino acids as animal foods do, only in differing amounts? As long as you are getting enough calories from a healthy diet, eating plant foods will give you all the amino acids you need, by themselves or in combination with one another."

The foods listed below are considered complete proteins, meaning they contain all of the essential amino acids:

- Nuts
- Soy foods, such as tofu, tempeh, miso, and soy milk
- Sprouted seeds – each type of sprout has differing proportions of nutrients, so it's best to eat a variety of them
- Grains, especially amaranth and quinoa, are highest in protein and are high-quality proteins
- Beans and legumes, especially when eaten raw
- Spirulina and chlorella (blue-green algae), which are over 60 percent protein

## Other Common Sources of Essential Amino Acids

You hear that you need to consume essential amino acids, but no one ever tells you what exactly they are. I have created the list below so you know some of the common essential amino acids and what foods provide them. You probably didn't even know you were getting them just by eating fruits and vegetables.

Histidine: Apple, pomegranates, alfalfa, beets, carrots, celery, cucumber, dandelion, endive, garlic, radish, spinach, turnip greens.

Arginine:  Alfalfa, beets, carrots, celery, cucumbers, green vegetables, leeks, lettuce, potatoes, radishes, parsnips, nutritional yeast.

Valine:  Apples, almonds, pomegranates, beets, carrots, celery, dandelion greens, lettuce, okra, parsley, parsnips, squash, tomatoes, turnips, nutritional yeast.

Tryptophan:  Alfalfa, Brussels sprouts, carrots, celery, chives, dandelion greens, endive, fennel, snap beans, spinach, turnips, nutritional yeast.

Threonine: Papayas, alfalfa sprouts, carrots, green leafy vegetables such as celery, collards, kale, and lettuce (especially iceberg), lima beans, laver (nori—a sea vegetable).

Phenylalanine:  Apples, pineapples, beets, carrots, parsley, spinach, tomatoes, nutritional yeast.

Methionine:  Apples, pineapples, brazil nuts, filberts, Brussels sprouts, cabbage, cauliflower, chives, dock (sorrel), garlic, horseradish, kale, watercress.

Lysine:  Apples, apricots, grapes, papayas, pears, alfalfa, beets, carrots, celery, cucumber, dandelion greens, parsley, spinach, turnip greens.

Leucine:  Avocados, papayas, olives, coconut, sunflower seeds.

Isoleucine:  Egg whites, soy protein, chicken, turkey, fish, seaweed, lamb.

## Fibrous Carbohydrates

One of my favorite memories I have of my Grandma Marion was the love she had for her garden in her backyard. It was full of vegetables and I can remember her saying the joys of life came from all the green vegetables she planted. She would talk about her garden daily and I often wondered what she meant by the joys of life. One day I asked my grandmother, "What does 'the joy of life' mean?" She said, "Baby, it means you will live a longer and healthier life if you eat more green than any other color." The coolest thing was you could eat as much as you like and never gain weight. Little did any of us know growing up that eating green would become a vegan lifestyle! The Power of 14 is not a vegan program but it does ask that you consume everything green as you go through your journey.

So what are the benefits of eating green? "Researchers from the Walters + Eliza Hall Institute of Medical Research in Australia found that innate lymphoid cells, which are a kind of immune cell, promote good intestinal health by keeping 'bad' bacteria out of the intestine, and helping to control or prevent conditions like bowel cancer, food allergy and inflammatory disease." I'm no doctor, but I do believe eating green keeps the doctor away.

## Fats

Fat:     There are two main sources of fat – animal and vegetable. There are three main types of fat – saturated, monounsaturated, and polyunsaturated. Saturated fats have a high impact on the development of increased blood cholesterol levels, whereas monounsaturated and polyunsaturated fats tend to lower blood cholesterol levels. The function of fat is to protect the vital organs of the body and to provide heat and energy. Certain fats also supply certain vitamins.

Saturated Fat: This type of fat tends to have a marked effect on raising blood cholesterol levels and is most often found in lard and animal fats.

Cholesterol: Cholesterol is a waxy, fat-like substance that is present in all body tissues, and is essential for normal body functions. The body manufactures all the cholesterol needs, but as cholesterol is found in many foods that we eat, diet can contribute to an overabundance of cholesterol in the body. If it becomes excessive in the bloodstream, it can contribute to the development of fatty deposits on the inner linings of the arteries and can lead to a heart attack.

## Do you know that...?

1. Not all calories are created equal; when your body uses them, for instance, the body turns food fat into body fat more rapidly than protein or carbohydrates.
2. People with a higher percentage of body fat tend to crave more fatty foods.
3. Americans eat an average of 6 lbs of potatoes each year – about 870 grams of fat or 58 tablespoons of oil for each person in this country. That means we consume 1.5 billion pounds of potato chips a year.
4. A small order of fast-food fries contains approximately 12 grams of fat.
5. Fish is very lean and only swims in water. Adding butter and dressings makes your fish dish high in fat.
6. In order to keep your salad healthy, skip the dressing. Adding just two tablespoons of regular high-fat salad dressing makes your salad contain as much fat as a hamburger. Just one tablespoon of regular salad dressing can contain 6 to 9 grams of fat – about as much as two pats of margarine or butter.
7. When choosing between a donut or two slices of whole-wheat bread or a bagel, skip the donut. Calories from fatty foods are more likely to be stored as fat than those from

protein or carbohydrate. Meaning the donut is more likely to "settle on your hips."

8.  Better to choose lean roast beef over a hamburger. It will contain less fat.

## Salt vs. Sodium

What is the difference between Salt and Sodium?

Sodium is needed mainly to maintain the blood volume, blood pressure, and water balance in the body. Consuming too much sodium in one's diet can cause high blood pressure. Consuming too much sodium and salt in one's diet can also lead to weight gain.

Salt and sodium are interchangeable, yet salt and sodium are not the same thing. Sodium, which is found naturally in most foods, accounts for approximately 40% of table salt. Therefore, when salt is added to food, the sodium content increases by approximately 40% of the amount of salt added. Keeping it to the point: If you are on the Power of 14 plan, understand all processed foods in a package or jar are high in sodium and are out of the question (tomato sauce, soups, pickles, sauerkraut, cured meats, bologna, salami, hot dogs, sausage, processed cheeses, salty snacks, all condiments such as ketchup, mayonnaise, and salad dressing). Like Smokey the Bandit always says in case of a fire, "Stop, drop, and roll." Meaning run to the kitchen right this minute and throw all of this out of your house. What are you waiting for?

## Sugar

Sugar is killing our society. It is just as addictive as street drugs. Yet it is used so often because it is one of the easiest ways to make something taste a lot better. Just think of a coffee or latte; we add sugar or flavoring (sugar) to sweeten to our liking.

I can remember as a kid coming home after school to make

the warmest and easiest thing ever created: bread with butter and lots of sugar on it. I remember warming up the stove and making half the bread loaf for the boys. Yummy! Looking at it now, I wonder how we didn't show signs such as diabetes, high uric acid, obesity, heart disease, hypertension, stroke, kidney disease, and other conditions.

As a society today, kids as well as adults overindulge in sugar. The more you intake, the more you want. The problem is that it is hidden in many of the foods we consume on a daily basis. These foods should be avoided at all cost. The majority of refined carbohydrates and sugars lurk in the form of wheat and sugar. Unless the ingredient list states "whole wheat," assume it is made with refined wheat. White rice is another popular refined carbohydrate; instead if you are looking for a better choice, choose brown rice or wild rice.

I have listed some more foods to help you out. These foods contain sugar in one form or another. Common food items include bread, pasta, crackers, cookies, muffins, cakes, boxed cereals, frozen treats, pretzels, soda, and other sugar-sweetened beverages and candy. Instead look for whole-grain breads, baked goods, pastas, and snacks. The 41 agent says......Beware of "ose; it is a synonym for sugar, such as high fructose corn syrup, cane juice, malt syrup, and any word ending in "ose," such as glucose, fructose, etc. Knowing what's in your foods will help you to win!

Make a plan and follow through with it. Your life depends on it. Make it a great life by taking control of all the bad food choices you have ever made. The Power of 14 will keep you on track. Burn it hard! – #41

# Testimonial from Maureen

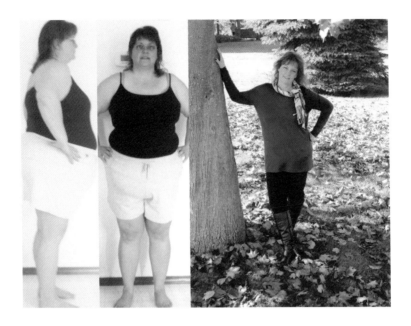

In 2008, my daughter left our hometown to go to WWU in Bellingham, WA. She had some difficulties adjusting, and began to put on weight. I was watching a TV show, and a story came on about Anthony McClanahan and his 41 Sports Fitness program. It looked like a lot of fun, so I found the clip on the Internet, and sent it to my daughter. She didn't say too much about it, but she watched it, and called Anthony. She started working with him, and before I knew it, she had lost a lot of weight, and was healthy and strong. She graduated from the University of Washington, and moved back home to plan her wedding. She began to put the weight back on, panicked, and called Anthony. She put together a group of people who wanted to workout for a weekend, and Anthony came to our town and ran a weekend boot camp for the group; I was part of the group. When I met him, I weighed 275 pounds. Believe it or not, I had lost weight, about ten pounds, before he came to town.

The group eventually fell apart, but I kept working out, working with Anthony all along. He sent me e-mails with workouts. He sent me phone text messages all day, every day. He sent me daily menus to follow. He worked with me to pick out foods that would work with my health issues (I am hypothyroid). I was "pre"-diabetic. I was scared.

Anthony kept on me, encouraging me. He would call me to encourage me. I kept working out, kept eating right. At the beginning of 2013, I resolved to lose 100 pounds. It was a daunting thought, but I knew I could do it if I only worked hard. The daily encouragement and motivation was wonderful. By the end of 2013, I had lost 80 pounds. I didn't reach my goal (yet!), but Anthony didn't give up on me. As a matter of fact, he was very encouraging, calling me when I was down, telling me I was doing great.

Thanks, Anthony! I have a way to go yet, maybe another 30–40 pounds, but I will get there with his help.

*A note from your trainer:*
*In your first 14 days, please follow the*
*Power of 14 plan exactly how it reads*
*before you start eating any of these foods listed.*

# 14 Supplements
## (vitamins and minerals that will
## fire up your fat-burning program)

These are supplements and vitamins 41
uses daily to keep his 43-year-old body in
top shape! When taking any supplements or
vitamins, always consult with your doctor first.

~ #41

Whey protein – As a result of cheese production, the byproduct is a liquid material composed of a mix of globular proteins. Studies have been conducted on rodents; these preclinical studies suggest that whey protein may contain anti-inflammatory and/or anticancer properties. More research is currently being conducted because the ways in which they support human health have piqued an interest in scientists, including a possibility of treating several diseases. More information on whey protein can be found on medicalnewstoday.com; just search "Whey Protein."

Soy protein – Soy is a plant-based protein that comes from soybeans. Like whey, it is considered a complete protein and contains all the essential amino acids. While whey is rich in the branch-chained amino acids, soy is rich in both arginine and glutamine. Arginine helps muscle formation. Soy has a slower absorption rate than whey, which means it takes the body longer to digest the protein. Therefore, soy is less helpful in rebuilding muscle, but extremely helpful in forming new muscle tissue. Because soy is plant based, it is a great alternative to whey protein for those dealing with dairy allergies.

There are some concerns about the isoflavones found in soy. Studies suggest that isoflavones can disrupt the body's hormonal balance. As a result soy intake is sometimes implicated in thyroid problems and changes in testosterone and estrogen levels. Also, some of the inhibitors found in soy have been known to obstruct digestion.

Plant protein – A diet low in carbohydrates and high in plant-based proteins could improve blood cholesterol levels while promoting weight loss, according to a new study. True fact: Saturated fats can cause cardiovascular disease and type 2 diabetes. If your diet is rich in saturated fats (found mostly in meat, dairy, and eggs), you are more likely to suffer from heart disease in the years to come. Unsaturated fats (found in nuts and seeds) are the alternative and help to keep your heart healthy.

Along with the protein I like to take, here is the list to complete my favorite 14 supplements and vitamins. I've included different foods that you can eat anytime to continue on your fat-fighting journey; they also help in building your immune system.

L. Glutamine – Free-range eggs, Chicken, Bison
Vitamin C – Broccoli, Brussels sprouts, Bell peppers
Krill oil – Source of omega 3
Flax seed oil – Flax seeds, Source of omega 3
Magnesium – Quinoa, Chickpeas, Tuna, Almonds
Selenium – Tuna, Halibut, Chicken, Oats
Zinc – Salmon, Pine nuts, Pumpkin seeds, Lobster, Clams
B6 – Turkey, Winter squash, Salmon
B12 – Sardines, Lamb, Cod
Garlic – Garlic also has Vitamin C, B6, Magnesium, and Selenium
Chromium picolinate – Tomatoes, Onions, Romaine lettuce

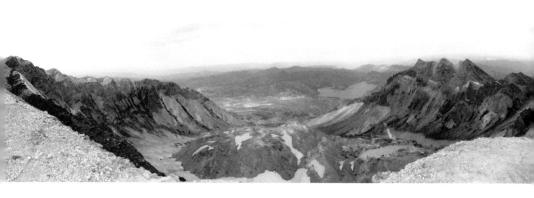

*Drive Hard to the Top! – #41*

# 14 "Energy" Foods That Will Supercharge Your Body!

The world we live in is full of pollutants in the air we breathe, and additives in the foods we eat. In order to fight against that which has become our natural environment, we must eat healthy to rid our bodies of the toxins that otherwise would build up. Since most people never really have an eating plan, they tend to eat what is fast and convenient. Without a plan, it is hard to eat right. Therefore I have listed 14 Power Foods to help you kick-start your metabolism and help you get back on the playing field faster. We are all looking for a healthier and leaner body. By eating these foods you are well on your way.

We all know the story of Friday Night Lights; every Friday night, high school football players all over the United States prepare to battle against one another to win the rights of the number one team in their area. The one thing that most people don't understand is the variety of foods that are needed to nourish the body. Grandma Marion knew this and the nutrition we received helped us to achieve optimal performance. She fed us every Friday before the game with the vegetables from her garden. Grandma made sure that we all ate our vegetables! Grandma, thank you for the Power of 14.

Grapefruit – High in Fiber
Kiwi – High in Fiber
Lemon – Vitamin C

Lentils – Iron
Green cabbage – Cruciferous vegetables
Asparagus – Folate
Green peppers – Vitamin C
Mustard greens – Vitamin C
Spinach – High in Iron
Cauliflower – Cruciferous vegetables
Broccoli – Cruciferous vegetables
Sweet potatoes – Vitamin A
Blueberries – Vitamin A
Carrots – Vitamin A

# 14 Creative Ways to Simplify Your Plan

No one ever said following a food plan would be easy. I will say that what you put into your plan is what you will get out of it. The Power of 14 is not a diet, it is simply an eating plan to help you change your lifestyle and eating habits. In the end, you will feel better, look better, and have a better lifestyle. The side-effect is you will shed weight. Looking at all the testimonials in this book, each person had a different issue they encountered. Some had major weight to drop and some had health issues to deal with. The bottom line is that they dealt with the problem by following the plan exactly how it was written.

The 14 steps that I am about to tell you are very important for you to follow in order to ensure success with the Power of 14. Following these steps will make your journey a bit easier to maintain and handle.

#1    Go inside your fridge and pantries and throw away or donate every boxed good, canned food, processed food, salt, sodium, sugar, and yeast products you can find. Say good-bye to your "diet" drinks as well. Set Go!

#2    What's your weight? GO and get your starting weight and only weigh again after a week.

#3    On Sunday, pick up your shopping list and go to the store. Try to go early as this will help you in getting into a schedule. Every Sunday begin with a new plan.

#4    At the store, buy only what is on your list. If you stick to the list, you won't pick up things you don't need.

#5    Buy only green fruits until the program suggests you eat other colors. Remember, the brighter the color the more sugar it has.

#6    Prepare all your foods on Sunday and again on Thursday. Cut up chicken and bag other meats in ziplock bags. Cut up all vegetables and package in bags to last you a few days. On Thursday, you will need to go back to the store for more veggies or maybe they will last till Sunday.

#7    Place small bags of chicken to cook up in the freezer. Never use a microwave as it takes out all the nutrients. Place in an oven or even cook as many cut-up breasts as you can and place in freezer or fridge to reheat. Boiling and barbecuing work as well.

#8    Eggs are essential for protein. We eat only the white in this program. Boil a couple dozen and place in the fridge. If you are only eating 6–9 in a week, boil only what you need. Guys will need more protein than women. Make sure to figure out how much protein you need by reading the protein section: "How to Calculate Your Protein Needs."

#9    After putting all of your foods together for the week, it is now time to organize your supplements and vitamins. If you're not taking any, it's okay. This plan can be completed without taking them. I always say a protein shake is an extra meal and is a lifesaver when you can't find food. Place protein powder in 2 shaker cups and sit out for morning, then all you have to do is add water and drink. Take the other to work or keep in your car with a bottle of water. Planning is essential to success. Find a vitamin tray, or small fishing tackle box works great to separate vitamins.

#10   Following the plan is key. Be sure to eat and drink every

2.5 hours of your day. I have online clients that have never met me and every 2.5 hours for the first 30 days, I send out a text to eat 4 to 6 times per day. This gets them in a routine. No excuse, you must eat to lose weight. You must drink fluids to be able to speed up your metabolism. Metabolism is essentially the speed at which our body's motor is running. The speed at which our body burns calories is called the metabolic rate. It's how fast your "motor" is running when you're still in a reclined position or sleeping. About 60–75% of energy is expended by the body at rest in such activities.

#11    Let's not make this program the highlight of our day. What I mean is, don't let it be the only exciting thing you've done all day long. Try to not think about the plan and make it as routine as possible. Some people will have a hard time not eating something with sugar in it or ordering a coffee with cream in it as they normally do daily. This is change, and for most humans change is difficult. Each day must be a new day. Take each one as if you were on a professional football team preparing to play a new team each week. Find your bubble and go for it. The journal is a tool that will help you stay focused.

#12    Journal time: Start YOUR journal! Take the time at each meal or at least at the end of your day to record how you are feeling, your struggles, and your successes. If you need extra support, set up a blog or document on your computer to help you begin your journal. If you want online support, please visit my website at www.powerof14.com for information.

#13    Finding your bubble will keep your mind clear and free of any non-believers that do not think you will succeed. Family, friends, and coworkers tend to not be very supportive until they have seen results. Finding your bubble can keep your mind right. Find it and conquer it. The only person you see when you wake up in the morning is you. Conquer the Power of 14 and win.

#14    As long as you have a plan and a little help, this program will work. Find a driven person close to you and share your daily experience. As a trainer, I like to know what the client is feeling daily. I ask that you train daily and eat from the plan. As much as I would like to talk more on the types of training you should do to take weight off, I will say that with this plan, 15 to 20 minutes a day in a boot-camp-style program is enough to keep you losing between 2 and 6 pounds per week. You must follow the plan exactly as it reads.

# Blue Print to Excellence: 14 Weight Loss Metabolism Boosting Dishes

To win we must plan.
To plan we must have a coach.
The Power of 14 is your food
coach to success.
Follow the plan and win! ~ #41

# 14 Simple Metabolism-Boosting Dishes by 41

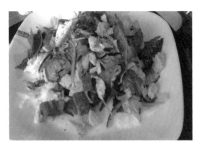

### 1. The 41 Anytime Salad
Green salad
Green pepper
Cucumber
Spinach
Onion
Grilled chicken
Add lemon juice

### 2. 41 Tuna Salad Blast
Can tuna in water only or fresh.
Avocado
Bell peppers
Egg whites
Lemon juice
Serve with cucumbers…no bread!

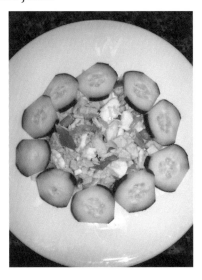

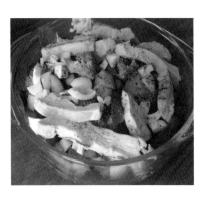

### 3. 41 Chicken Breast Delight Salad
Chicken breast, baked or barbecued
Egg whites
Baby tomatoes
Sliced avocado
Broccoli
Green and yellow pepper
Cucumber

## 4. 41 Protein Pancake

1 cup of minute Quaker oats (small oats)
3 egg whites
Almond milk to moisten
Add cinnamon to your liking.
Makes 1–2 pancakes.
Skillet on medium heat
Olive oil in pan
Grapefruit. We drizzle some of the juice on ours.
Optional: with honey and add blueberries

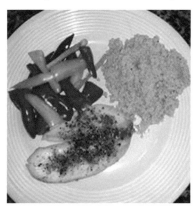

## 5. The Field Is on Fire

Tilapia
Quinoa
Red and yellow peppers

## 6. The Green Bandit

(Can be used to top any meal.)
2 poblano peppers
2 green chili peppers
1 red onion
Roast all together.
Peel skin off peppers.
Put all in blender with a handful of cilantro.
Olive oil to thin it
Blend well.

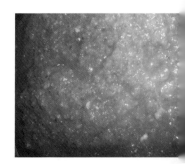

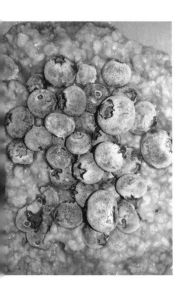

## 7. Oatmeal
Blueberries
Cinnamon
Honey

## 8. 41 Halibut
Onion
Spinach
Broccoli
Quinoa
Sliced green apple on the side
Lemon to taste

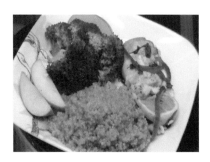

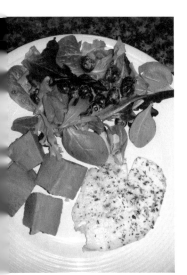

## 9. The 41 Power Play
Turkey breast (1)
with Italian seasoning & freeze-dried dill
Baby spring lettuce
20 blueberries
1/2 sweet potato

## 10. Quinoa Touchdown
Chicken
Asparagus
Broccoli
Cabbage
Yellow pepper

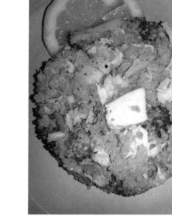

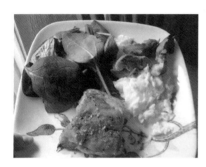

## 11. 41 Savory's Salmon
Sweet potatoes
Avocado
Spinach

## 12. Asparagus and Lemon

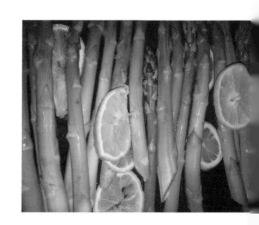

### 13. 41 Veggie Wrap
2–4 egg whites
Avocado
Green bell peppers

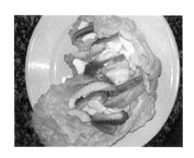

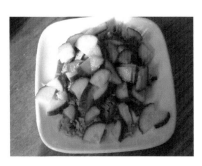

### 14. Tuna and Cucumbers
Lemon juice

# Testimonial from Sandy

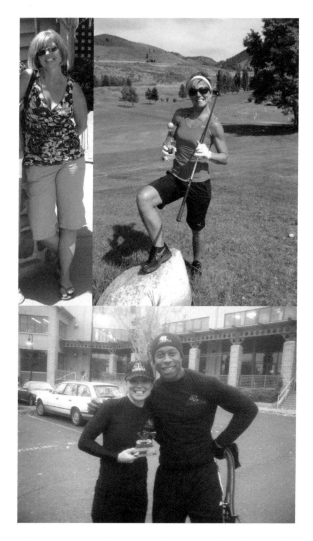

When I first met Anthony, whom I fondly call Mac, I was watching a high school basketball game and one of my girlfriends suggested that I join his boot camp. My response was that it sounded like fun, but that I had better get in shape before I jumped into his rigorous exercise routine. Mac heard and responded with,

"That is silly! You just need to show up Monday and let me help you reach your goals!" True to his word, Mac delivered. That was five years ago. I lost thirty-five pounds in the first four months, increased my cardio fitness, and strengthened my body beyond my expectations. The five-plus days a week, year-round outdoor boot-camp style training in every kind of Pacific Northwest weather, innovative training methods, ongoing motivational messages, and his Power of 14 food plan made it all possible.

As a former high school and club sport athlete, jazzercise junkie, and long-distance bicyclist, staying slim, healthy, and strong were attributes that I valued in myself. However, it had been a long time since physical fitness and nutrition were a consistent part of my life and I was left to suffer with a chronic pain in my shoulder and a chubby weak body. Although I didn't like it, I had resigned myself to my aging and changing 45-year middle-aged mom physique. Through my new life's journey with Mac, I now know how wrong I was. Mac taught me how to regain my physical toughness, encouraging me all the way to push harder, run faster, rise to any challenge, and feed my body like it deserved. The weight came off, which was the most obvious and a wonderful result of all of my hard work along with Mac's training and nutritional guidance. After the "hundreds" of pushups, triceps and shoulder strengthening exercises, my pains are a distant memory. But the transformation goes much further than physical. I am mentally stronger than I have ever been and I have a renewed confidence and pride in myself.

Along with my exercise routine, I implemented Mac's Power of 14 food plan, which became the key to my immediate weight loss and what continues my maintenance today. Through his educational pointers, I purged my home of nonessential foods and those fatty sauce-laden casserole recipes that I was raised on. Shopping for groceries transitioned into spending the majority of my time in the produce and lean protein departments to no longer wandering up and down every aisle selecting prepackaged processed foods. While learning to cook with fresh and pure ingredients, I have enjoyed meals bursting with natural flavors. I keep Mac's Power of 14 food plan in the front of my recipe book and central to my meal planning process.

41 Sports Fitness Boot Camps have also become a family activity. My husband and daughter, when she's home from college; join in the boot camps with Mac. People always ask me if the workouts ever get easier and my response is, not if you are fully committed and challenging yourself, which is never a problem with Mac. He always makes boot camp fun and encourages us to test our mental and physical strength by entering fun-runs and other physical fitness events. I even placed first in my age division at a regional obstacle mud run!

Over the past five years I have definitely continued to maintain my dedication to health and fitness with Mac. Though, on those occasions where I feel like I have gotten a bit lazy in the nutrition piece, Mac is there to encourage me to get back on track with the Power of 14, sometimes subtly and other times not so subtly, but always with care. Through it all there is one special characteristic of Mac that he's exemplified from the first day I met him. It's been said that "No one cares what you know, unless they know that you care." That is Mac. He cares very much for me and my boot camp "sisters and brothers" beyond measure. Not only is Mac my trainer, he is my friend and one of the most important people in my life. He has welcomed me into his 41 Sports family, supports me in all of my efforts, and celebrates my accomplishments as I continue in my life's fitness journey.

I am forever 41 Sports strong!

Sandy Thomas

# Power of 14 Journal

By using the journal provided in the "14 Days of Success," you can track your progress daily to help you celebrate your successes and track your challenges. This will also give you an opportunity to set small goals daily based on the successes and challenges. By keeping a journal it will keep you honest, as if you had 41 as your personal food coach. It will give you a place to record information needed later when developing your 3rd and 4th quarter weeks. Please write in your journal daily. Write some goals for the day. Did you miss a meal? Were you on target? Did you get a compliment for changing your eating habits? Write anything in your journal that will help keep you on track. Stay positive and win.

# The Power of 14
# Shopping List

*A shopping list in which you can eat from anytime you get hungry.*

I have created a shopping list of foods to get you started. For your first week of eating, please stick to these foods listed on this page. The 2nd week you will be able to add more of the power foods and then move into the proteins. I have made some notes and it's now time to enter the bubble.

Note: You don't like chicken; eat fish instead. Surely, we would never want you to eat something you don't like. Some people may have allergic reactions to different types of meat. It may be easier to keep meats out of your daily program. Not a problem – you will just have to look at the protein list for another source. Be sure to write in your journal what works for you.

The war on Abs is won in the kitchen.
Set Go! ~ #41

# Shopping List – Week 1

| Foods | Sodium Free |
|---|---|
| Egg whites- (Protein) | Eggplant |
| Oatmeal- (Protein) | Summer Squash |
| Protein shakes-(Protein) | Cucumbers |
| Grapefruit- (Fiber) | Bell Peppers |
| Kiwi- (Fiber) | Mushrooms |
| Almonds- (Protein) | Apples (Green) |
| Quinoa- (Protein) | |
| Romaine Lettuce - (Fiber- Vitamin A) | **Meats** |
| Green Cabbage-(Vitamin C) | Turkey (lean) |
| Asparagus- (Pantohenic acid- Calcium) | Chicken |
| Lentils-(Folate) | Fish |
| Mustard greens-(Folate) | No Red meats |
| Spinach-(Folate) | |
| Cauliflower- (Vitamin C) | **Don't Forget to eat** |
| Kale-(Folate) | Water |
| Broccoli-(Vitmain C) | Green Tea |
| Sweet potatoes-(Vitamin A) | Caffeine |
| Blueberries-(Fiber) | Cinnamon |
| Tomatoes-(Potassium) | Lemons/Lemon Juice |
| Lemons-(Vitamin C) | No Salt Seasoning |

# 14 Days to Success – Week 1

**Only eat the foods from week one's shopping list.**

You are now on the Power of 14. Please notice some of the lifestyle changes listed below.

Remember this is a lifestyle change, NOT A FAD DIET. The journey will be long and hard. As long as you remember to find your bubble, the plan will go smoothly. Drive hard to the top!

If you would like to make a wrap, you may use lettuce or green spinach tortilla wraps.

No fruit, unless it is listed.

No dairy or bread of any kind.

No sugar added to anything.

Use "No Salt" seasonings only.

Green vegetables for snacks or protein shakes.

If you get hungry, drink a shake. You can also eat from the shopping list if you need a quick meal and stray away from selected meal of the day. Try to eat proteins and cruciferous veggies.

Please don't forget to stock up on vitamins and supplements.

Suggested supplements can be purchased at www.powerof14. com

41's number-one choice for supplements is: Prograde.

Did you know if your body gives off more heat, you increase your metabolism? When you increase your metabolism, you burn more calories. To help make this happen you can add hot peppers to your foods to increase your body temperature, which will help you burn fat faster. Some recommended peppers are:

- Habaneras
- Cayenne Chiles
- Jalapenos

Let the journey begin. You have shopped for the essentials and now it's time to begin the journey:

Did you prep for the week? If you are only cooking for one day, stop and go back to the beginning. We must make a plan and follow it through. Your success comes from your ability to have follow-through skills. Bring each moment of your day as if it were your last.

Set Go!
"Many times in life we walk down roads in
complete darkness.
The Power of 14 is the light you have been
looking for."
Drive hard to the top! – #41

# 14 Days to Success – Week 1

### 4 weeks = 4 quarters

Note: Always take your vitamins. It's your safety net. If you miss out on eating a meal, your vitamins and supplements will replenish your system for the day.

### Day 1

**Wake up:** Green tea and lemon juice

**Breakfast:** Protein shake with spinach
½ cup blueberries
$H_2O$ or almond milk (plain) Ice

**Snack:** Cucumbers and white chicken breast
Only half breast
Cook boiled or baked

**Lunch:** 2 cups green salad or spinach
Add ½-can tuna plain
Lemon juice

**Snack:** Protein shake

**Dinner:** 1 cup steamed broccoli mixed in quinoa
Small green salad with lemon juice on top

At night if you get hungry, it's okay to have a single scoop of protein in water.

## Journal: How did you do at each meal?

Breakfast: _____
_____
_____
_____

Snack: _____
_____
_____
_____

Lunch: _____
_____
_____
_____

Snack: _____
_____
_____
_____

Dinner: _____
_____
_____
_____

What was the biggest challenge of the day?
_____
_____
_____

What is your goal for tomorrow?
_____
_____
_____

Write how you did overall in your journal:
_____
_____
_____

# Day 2

Wake up:  Green tea and lemon juice

**Breakfast:**  8 oz cooked oatmeal mix in cinnamon and
1 tsp of honey
1 Grapefruit
½ cup of almond milk

**Snack:**  Protein shake

**Lunch:**  3 oz white-meat tuna packed in water
2 cups green salad
1/8 avocado (2 tbsp)
Lemon juice

**Snack:**  Less than 20 almonds

**Dinner:**  4 oz grilled white meat chicken breast
1 small sweet potato
1 cup steamed spinach
Small green salad with lemon juice on top

Journal:  How did you do at each meal?

Breakfast: _____
_____
_____
_____

Snack: _____
_____
_____
_____

Lunch: _____
_____
_____
_____

Snack: _____
_____
_____
_____

Dinner: _____
_____
_____
_____

What was the biggest challenge of the day?
_____
_____
_____

What is your goal for tomorrow?
_____
_____
_____

Write how you did overall in your journal:
_____
_____
_____

# Day 3

**Wake up:** Green tea and lemon juice

**Breakfast:** 2–3 egg whites wrapped in lettuce
(take all of your vitamins for the morning)
Fluid up.

**Snack:** Protein shake – only add water

**Lunch:** 2 cups green salad or spinach
Add half chicken breast
Squeeze lemon juice on top

**Snack:** Broccoli mixed with cucumbers

**Dinner:** White fish of choice (steamed, baked, or barbecued)
Quinoa, 2/3 cup
Small green salad with lemon juice on top

Journal:  How did you do at each meal?

Breakfast: _____
_____
_____
_____

Snack: _____
_____
_____
_____

Lunch: _____
_____
_____
_____

Snack: _____
_____
_____
_____

Dinner: _____
_____
_____
_____

What was the biggest challenge of the day?
_____
_____
_____

What is your goal for tomorrow?
_____
_____
_____

Write how you did overall in your journal:
_____
_____
_____

# Day 4

Wake up: Green tea and lemon juice

Breakfast: 2–3 egg whites wrapped in lettuce (take all of your vitamins for the morning)
Fluid up.

Snack: Protein shake – only add water

Lunch: 4 oz lean turkey
2 cups green vegetables salad
Top with lemon juice

Snack: Cauliflower steamed or raw

Dinner: 4 oz grilled white meat
Broccoli
Green salad with lemon juice

Journal: How did you do at each meal?

Breakfast: _____
_____
_____
_____

Snack: _____
_____
_____
_____

Lunch: _____
_____
_____
_____

Snack: _____
_____
_____
_____

Dinner: _____
_____
_____
_____

What was the biggest challenge of the day?
_____
_____
_____

What is your goal for tomorrow?
_____
_____
_____

Write how you did overall in your journal:
_____
_____
_____

# Day 5

Wake up:  Green tea and lemon juice

Breakfast:  Oatmeal, honey, cinnamon

Snack:  Broccoli mixed with cucumbers

Lunch:  Protein shake with water

Snack:  15 almonds

Dinner:  Chicken breast salad
Sliced almonds on top and lemon juice

Journal:  How did you do at each meal?

Breakfast: _____
_____
_____
_____

Snack: _____
_____
_____
_____

Lunch: _____
_____
_____
_____

Snack: _____
_____
_____
_____

Dinner: _____
_____
_____
_____

What was the biggest challenge of the day?
_____
_____
_____

What is your goal for tomorrow?
_____
_____
_____

Write how you did overall in your journal:
_____
_____
_____

# Day 6

**Wake up:** Green tea and lemon juice

**Breakfast:** Oatmeal, honey, cinnamon
1 chopped green apple

**Snack:** Protein shake

**Lunch:** White-meat tuna wraps
Mix olive oil or flaxseed oil in your tuna. Add lemon juice
and eat plain or wrap in lettuce. You can also cut half an
avocado to mix in your tuna. Never use mayonnaise again.
Try your tuna with green bell peppers.

**Snack:** Protein shake

**Dinner:** Half chicken breast
1 medium sweet potato
1 cup steamed string beans

## Journal: How did you do at each meal?

Breakfast: _____
_____
_____
_____

Snack: _____
_____
_____
_____

Lunch: _____
_____
_____
_____

Snack: _____
_____
_____
_____

Dinner: _____
_____
_____
_____

What was the biggest challenge of the day?
_____
_____
_____

What is your goal for tomorrow?
_____
_____
_____

Write how you did overall in your journal:
_____
_____
_____

# Day 7

**Wake up:**  Green tea and lemon juice

**Breakfast:**  Egg whites
Spinach
Turkey scramble

**Snack:**  Protein shake with water

**Lunch:**  Sliced chicken breast
over a bed of greens
Add lemon juice on top

**Snack:**  20 almonds

**Dinner:**  Quinoa dish
Mix in chicken
Add green veggies

### Journal: How did you do at each meal?

Breakfast: _____
_____
_____
_____

Snack: _____
_____
_____
_____

Lunch: _____
_____
_____
_____

Snack: _____
_____
_____
_____

Dinner: _____
_____
_____
_____

What was the biggest challenge of the day?
_____
_____

What is your goal for tomorrow?
_____
_____

Write how you did overall in your journal:
_____
_____
_____

# Shopping List – Week 2

| Foods | Sodium Free |
|---|---|
| Egg whites- (Protein) | Eggplant |
| Cayenne Chiles-(Fiber- Vitamin A) | Summer Squash |
| Protein shakes-(Protein) | Cucumbers |
| Grapefruit- (Fiber) | Bell Peppers |
| Habaneras-(Capsaicin) | Mushrooms |
| Jalapenos-(Capsaicin- Vitamin C) | Apples (Green) |
| Quinoa- (Protein) | |
| Romaine Lettuce -(Fiber- Vitamin A) | **Meats** |
| Green Cabbage-(Vitamin C) | Turkey (lean) |
| Asparagus-(Pantohenic acid- Calcium) | Chicken |
| Lentils-(Folate) | Fish/Salmon |
| Mustard greens-(Folate) | No Red meats |
| Spinach-(Folate) | **Wild meat** |
| Cauliflower- (Vitamin C) | **Don't Forget to eat** |
| Kale-(Folate) | Water |
| Broccoli-(Vitamin C) | Green Tea |
| Avocado-(Potassium) | Caffeine |
| Blueberries-(Fiber) | Cinnamon |
| Yellow Bell Peppers- (B6- Folate- Vitamin C) | Lemons/Lemon Juice |
| Brussel Sprouts- (Vitamin C- Folate- Antioxidants) | No Salt Seasoning |

# 14 Days to Success – Week 2

**Only eat the foods from week two's shopping list**

So here we are in week two of food choices. It's time to climb farther up the mountain. We will follow the plan exactly as it asks and win. You ready? Make smart choices. You got this!

Reminders:

If you would like to make a wrap, you may use lettuce or green spinach tortilla wraps.

No fruit, unless it is listed.

No dairy or bread of any kind.

No sugar added to anything.

Use "No Salt" seasonings only.

Green vegetables for snacks or protein shakes.

If you get hungry, drink a shake. You can also eat from the shopping list if you need a quick meal and stray away from selected meal of the day. Try to eat proteins and cruciferous veggies.

Please don't forget to stock up on vitamins and supplements.

Suggested supplements can be purchased at www.powerof14. com

41's number-one choice for supplements is: Prograde.

Did you know if your body gives off more heat, you increase your metabolism? When you increase your metabolism, you burn more calories. To help make this happen you can add hot peppers to your foods to increase your body temperature, which will help you burn fat faster. Some recommended peppers are:

- Habaneras
- Cayenne chiles
- Jalapenos

*Set Go!*
*Never underestimate a weak mind.*
*It has full capability of taking control.*
*Feed it and watch it grow. – #41*

# 14 Days to Success – Week 2

Notes: Try and eat habaneras, cayenne chiles or jalapenos daily.

## Day 1

**Wake up:** Each morning when you wake up: Green tea and lemon juice

**Breakfast:** 8 oz of soy or almond milk
1 scoop lean protein
Handful of almonds mixed in blender. You can eat separate.

**Snack:** Green apple

**Lunch:** Chicken
2 cups green salad
Lemon juice

**Snack:** Green bell pepper – use honey if needed
Or a protein sports drink (fusion by prograde)
or lean protein powder in water

**Dinner:** Fish
1 cup steamed broccoli
Small green salad with lemon juice

## Journal:  How did you do at each meal?

Breakfast: _____
_____
_____
_____

Snack: _____
_____
_____
_____

Lunch: _____
_____
_____
_____

Snack: _____
_____
_____
_____

Dinner: _____
_____
_____
_____

What was the biggest challenge of the day?
_____
_____
_____

What is your goal for tomorrow?
_____
_____
_____

Write how you did overall in your journal:
_____
_____
_____

## Day Two

**Breakfast:** 1 cup soy or almond milk
1 scoop lean protein
Handful of almonds

**Snack:** Green apple

**Lunch:** 3 oz white-meat tuna packed in water
2 cups green salad
1/8 avocado mixed in tuna
Lemon juice

**Snack:** Protein shake or fusion

**Dinner:** 4 oz grilled white-meat chicken
1 cup steamed spinach
Small green salad with lemon juice

Journal:  How did you do at each meal?

Breakfast: _____
_____
_____
_____

Snack: _____
_____
_____
_____

Lunch: _____
_____
_____
_____

Snack: _____
_____
_____
_____

Dinner: _____
_____
_____
_____

What was the biggest challenge of the day?
_____
_____
_____

What is your goal for tomorrow?
_____
_____
_____

Write how you did overall in your journal:
_____
_____
_____

# Day Three

**Breakfast:** 4 egg whites
½ grapefruit

**Snack:** 1 scoop lean protein or fusion
Red bell pepper – use honey if needed

**Lunch:** Chicken
2 cups green vegetable
Salad with lemon juice

**Snack:** Green apple

**Dinner:** 4 oz grilled salmon
2/3 cup quinoa
1 cup steamed broccoli

**Snack:** Protein shake

### Journal: How did you do at each meal?

Breakfast: _____
_____
_____
_____

Snack: _____
_____
_____
_____

Lunch: _____
_____
_____
_____

Snack: _____
_____
_____
_____

Dinner: _____
_____
_____
_____

What was the biggest challenge of the day?
_____
_____
_____

What is your goal for tomorrow?
_____
_____
_____

Write how you did overall in your journal:
_____
_____
_____

# Day Four

**Breakfast:** Tuna wrapped in lettuce

**Snack:** Green apple

**Lunch:** Chicken breast
Small green salad with lemon juice

**Snack:** Green apple with cinnamon

**Dinner:** Turkey
12 steamed asparagus
Green salad with lemon juice

Journal: How did you do at each meal?

Breakfast: _____
_____
_____
_____

Snack: _____
_____
_____
_____

Lunch: _____
_____
_____
_____

Snack: _____
_____
_____
_____

Dinner: _____
_____
_____
_____

What was the biggest challenge of the day?
_____
_____
_____

What is your goal for tomorrow?
_____
_____
_____

Write how you did overall in your journal:
_____
_____
_____

# Day Five

**Breakfast:** Egg whites and grapefruit w/ cinnamon and honey
1 chopped green apple
Green tea

**Snack:** Protein shake

**Lunch:** 3 oz white-meat tuna (in water) lettuce wrap or
substitute with salmon (in water)
Add lemon juice inside wrap
2 cups mixed vegtables on the side

**Snack:** Protein shake
Green bell pepper – use honey if needed

**Dinner:** Chicken breast
1 medium sweet potato
1 cup steamed string beans

## Journal: How did you do at each meal?

Breakfast: _____
_____
_____
_____

Snack: _____
_____
_____
_____

Lunch: _____
_____
_____
_____

Snack: _____
_____
_____
_____

Dinner: _____
_____
_____
_____

What was the biggest challenge of the day?
_____
_____
_____

What is your goal for tomorrow?
_____
_____
_____

Write how you did overall in your journal:
_____
_____
_____

# Day Six

**Breakfast:** 4 egg whites
½ grapefruit

**Snack:** Handful of almonds
Sliced cucumber

**Lunch:** 2 cups torn spinach
Green veggies
4 oz sliced grilled chicken, add lemon juice

**Snack:** Protein shake

**Dinner:** 4 oz halibut (cooked)
2/3 cup blueberries
1 cup cooked zucchini
Small green salad with lemon juice

## Journal: How did you do at each meal?

Breakfast: _____
_____
_____
_____

Snack: _____
_____
_____
_____

Lunch: _____
_____
_____
_____

Snack: _____
_____
_____
_____

Dinner: _____
_____
_____
_____

What was the biggest challenge of the day?
_____
_____
_____

What is your goal for tomorrow?
_____
_____
_____

Write how you did overall in your journal:
_____
_____
_____

# Day Seven

**Breakfast:**  1 cup almond or soy milk
Protein shake

**Snack:**  Green apple

**Lunch:**  4 oz grilled salmon
2 cups green salad
1 whole carrot, chopped
Lemon juice

**Snack:**  Protein shake
Red bell pepper – use honey if needed

**Dinner:**  4 oz grilled white meat chicken
Steamed asparagus spears
Small green salad with lemon juice on top

## Journal: How did you do at each meal?

Breakfast: _____
_____
_____
_____

Snack: _____
_____
_____
_____

Lunch: _____
_____
_____
_____

Snack: _____
_____
_____
_____

Dinner: _____
_____
_____
_____

What was the biggest challenge of the day?
_____
_____
_____

What is your goal for tomorrow?
_____
_____
_____

Write how you did overall in your journal:
_____
_____
_____

Have fun, folks! Change up the types of fish you consume daily this week. If you would like to have chicken for lunch or dinner, simply switch meals for the day. Fish consumed should be salmon, tilapia, or cod. Baked, broiled, or barbecued. #41

The Power of 14 is truly the only way to accomplish your superior goals. You must follow your heart to reach the top. It has been 14 days and now it's time for you to check your weight. How did you do? I'm really proud of you for following the Power of 14 plan. Even though you are at the end of this book, know it's just the beginning to an adventure you'll never forget. Another two weeks of foods and journal writing awaits.

Set Go!
Enjoy the program, everyone.
Drive hard to the top and never look back!
#41, Anthony McClanahan

# Acknowledgements

Production Assistant: Tara Smyth
Photo Editor: Stacy Graves
Logo Design: David Vojo

Special thanks to Sandy Thomas, Erica Wayerski, Diana Hammond, Maureen Morgison, Ann Zink, Stacey Graves, Jamie Sziisz, Tim and Mandi Atkins, Ty Frederick, Lori Walton, Trina Funkhouser, and even though I listed Tara Smyth in the credits, I couldn't have finished this book to the end without her. She is 41 Sports Strong. Thank you to everyone who invested the many hours of following the plan and encouraging others to do the same. The Power of 14 is life changing. Drive hard to the top! ~ #41

# Sources

*Fresh Produce Guide* by Dr. Henry Richter, 2000

*Prescription for Nutritional Healing: A-to-Z Guide to Supplements*

Researchers from the Walters + Eliza Hall Institute of Medical Research in Australia

*Essential Amino Acids* by Thomas Stearns Lee, NMD

http://en.wikipedia.org/wiki/Whey_protein

http://www.fitday.com/fitness-articles/fitness/body-building/which-is-best-soy-protein-or-whey.html#b

http://www.naturodoc.com/library/nutrition/protein.htm

http://www.holistix.co.za/whey-protein-vs-soy-protein.html

CPSIA information can be obtained at www.ICGtesting.com
Printed in the USA
LVIW01n1106230215
427976LV00003B/6